The Ultimate Lean & Green Meat And Seafood Cookbook

Delicious Lean & Green Meat And Seafood Recipes For Beginners

Jesse Cohen

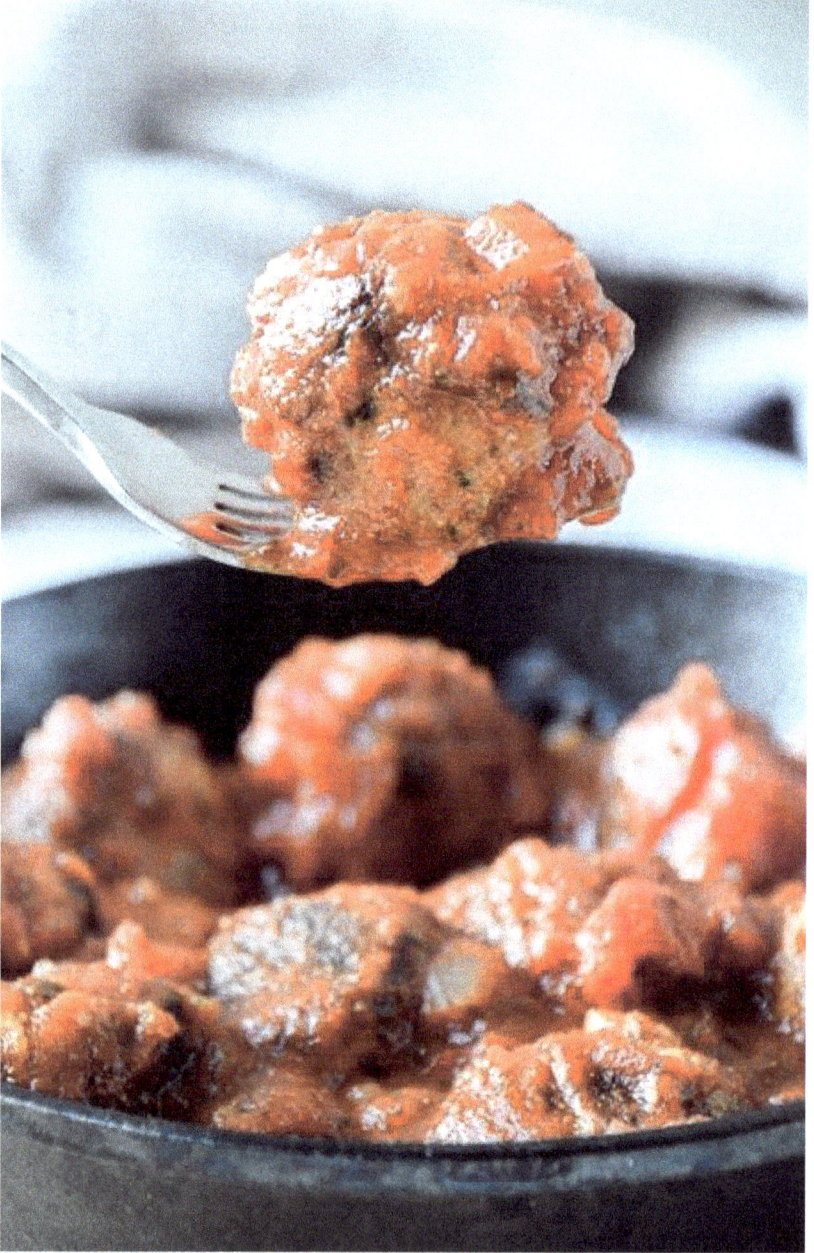

Table of contents

Chicken with Mushrooms

Servings: 4

Preparation Time: 15 minutes

Cooking Time: 20 minutes

Ingredients:

- 2 tablespoons of almond flour
- Salt and freshly ground black pepper, to taste
- 4 (4-ounce of) skinless, boneless chicken breasts
- 2 tablespoons of olive oil
- 6 garlic cloves, chopped
- ¾ pound fresh mushrooms, sliced
- ¾ cup of low-sodium chicken broth
- ¼ cup of balsamic vinegar
- 1 bay leaf
- ¼ teaspoon of dried thyme

Instructions:

1. In a bowl, mix together the flour, salt, and black pepper.
2. Coat the chicken breasts with flour mixture evenly.
3. In a skillet, heat the vegetable oil over medium-high heat and fry chicken for about 3 minutes.

4. Add the garlic and flip the chicken breasts.

5. Spread mushrooms over chicken and cook for about 3 minutes, shaking the skillet frequently.

6. Add the broth, vinegar, herb, and thyme and stir to mix.

7. Reduce the heat to medium-low and simmer, covered for about 10 minutes, flipping chicken occasionally.

8. With a slotted spoon, transfer the chicken onto a warm serving platter and with a bit of foil, cover to stay warm.

9. Place the pan of sauce over medium-high heat and cook, uncovered for about 7 minutes.

10. Remove the pan from heat and discard the herb.

11. Place sauce over chicken and serve hot.

Chicken with Broccoli

Servings: 4

Preparation Time: 15 minutes

Cooking Time: 22 minutes

Ingredients:

- 2 tablespoons of olive oil, divided
- 4 (4-ounce of) boneless, skinless chicken breasts, cut into small pieces
- Salt and freshly ground black pepper, to taste
- 1 onion, chopped finely
- 1 teaspoon of fresh ginger, grated
- 1 teaspoon of garlic, minced
- 1 cup of broccoli florets
- 1½ cups of fresh mushrooms, sliced
- 8 ounces of low-sodium chicken broth

Instructions:

1. In a large skillet, heat 1 tablespoon of oil over medium-high heat and fry the chicken pieces, salt, and black pepper for about 4-5 minutes or until golden brown.
2. With a slotted spoon, transfer the chicken onto a plate.

3. In the same skillet, heat the remaining oil over medium-high heat and sauté the onion, ginger, and garlic for about 4-5 minutes.

4. Add in mushrooms and cook for about 4-5 minutes, stirring frequently.

5. Add the broccoli and fry for about 3 minutes.

6. Add the cooked chicken and broth and fry for about 3-5 minutes

7. Add in the salt and black pepper and take away from the heat.

8. Serve hot.

Chicken & Veggies Stir Fry

Servings: 6

Preparation Time: 15 minutes

Cooking Time: 15 minutes

Ingredients:

- 2 tablespoons of fresh lime juice
- 2 tablespoons of fish sauce
- 1½ teaspoons of arrowroot starch
- 4 teaspoons of olive oil, divided
- 1-pound skinless, boneless chicken tenders, cubed
- 1 teaspoon of fresh ginger, minced
- 2 garlic cloves, minced
- ¾ teaspoon of red pepper flakes, crushed
- ¼ cup of water
- 4 cups of broccoli, cut into bite-sized pieces
- 3 cup of red bell pepper, seeded and sliced
- ¼ cup of pine nuts

Instructions:

1. In a bowl, add lemon juice, fish sauce, and arrowroot starch and blend until well combined. Set aside.

2. In a large non-stick sauté pan, heat 2 teaspoons of oil over high heat and cook chicken for about 6-8 minutes, stirring frequently.
3. Transfer the chicken into a bowl and put it aside.
1. 4 In an equivalent sauté pan, heat remaining oil over medium heat and sauté ginger, garlic, and red pepper
2. Flakes for about 1 minute.
3. 5 Add water, broccoli, and bell pepper and fry for about 2-3 minutes.
4. 6. Stir in chicken and juice mixture and cook for about 2-3 minutes.
5. 7. Stir in pine nuts and immediately remove from heat.
9. Serve hot.

Chicken & Broccoli Bake

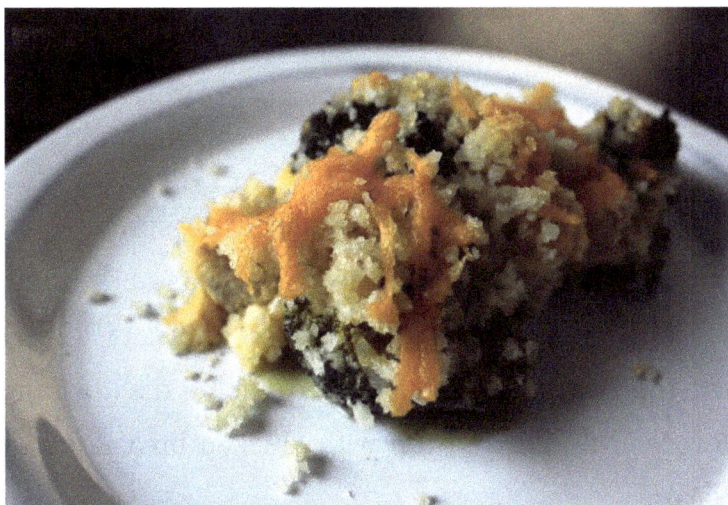

Servings: 6

Preparation Time: 15 minutes

Cooking Time: 24 minutes

Ingredients:

- Olive oil cooking spray
- 6 (6-ounce of) skinless, boneless chicken thighs
- 3 broccoli heads, cut into florets
- 4 garlic cloves, minced
- ¼ cup of extra-virgin olive oil
- 1 teaspoon of dried oregano, crushed

- 1 teaspoon of dried rosemary, crushed
- Salt and freshly ground black pepper, to taste

Instructions:

1. Preheat your oven to 375 degrees F.
2. Grease a large baking dish with cooking spray.
3. In a large bowl, add all the ingredients and toss to coat well.
4. At the bottom of the prepared baking dish, arrange the broccoli florets and top with chicken breasts in a single layer.
5. Bake for about 45 minutes.
6. Serve hot.

Cheesy Chicken & Spinach

Servings: 4

Preparation Time: 15 minutes

Cooking Time: 20 minutes

Ingredients:

- 2 tablespoons of olive oil, divided
- 4 (4-ounce of) boneless, skinless chicken thighs
- Salt and ground black pepper, as required
- 2 garlic cloves, minced
- 1 jalapeño pepper, chopped
- 10-ounce of frozen spinach, thawed
- 1/3 cup of low-fat Parmesan cheese, shredded

Instructions:

1. In a large skillet, heat 1 tablespoon of the oil over medium-high heat and cook the chicken with salt and black pepper for about 5-6 minutes per side.
2. Transfer the chicken into a bowl.
3. In the same skillet, heat the remaining oil over medium-low heat and sauté the garlic for about 1 minute.
4. Add the spinach and cook for about 1 minute.

5. Add the cheese, salt, and black pepper and stir to mix.
6. Spread the spinach mixture in the bottom of the skillet evenly.
7. Place chicken over spinach in a single layer.
8. Immediately adjust the heat to low and cook, covered for about 5 minutes.
9. Serve hot.

Chicken & Cauliflower Curry

Servings: 6

Preparation Time: 15 minutes

Cooking Time: 20 minutes

Ingredients:

- ¼ cup of olive oil
- 3 garlic cloves, minced
- 2 tablespoons of curry powder
- 1½ pounds skinless, boneless chicken thighs, cut into bite-sized pieces
- Salt and ground black pepper, as required
- 1-pound cauliflower, cut into small pieces
- 1 green bell pepper, seeded and chopped
- 14 ounces of unsweetened coconut milk
- ¼ cup of fresh parsley, chopped

Instructions:

1. In a large skillet, heat the oil over medium heat and sauté the garlic and chili powder for about 1 minute.
2. Add the chicken, salt, and black pepper and cook for about 5-6 minutes, stirring frequently.

3. With a slotted spoon, transfer the chicken onto a plate.
4. In the skillet, add the cauliflower and bell pepper and cook for about 2-3 minutes.
5. Add the coconut milk and simmer for about 5-7 minutes.
6. Stir in the cooked chicken, salt, and black pepper, and cook for about 2-3 minutes.
7. Serve hot with the garnishing of parsley.

Chicken & Veggies Casserole

Servings: 4

Preparation Time: 15 minutes

Cooking Time: 25 minutes

Ingredients:

- 1 tablespoon of olive oil
- 1 small onion, chopped
- 1 pepperoni pepper, seeded and sliced thinly
- ½ of red bell pepper, seeded and sliced thinly
- 2 teaspoons of garlic, minced
- 1 cup of fresh spinach, trimmed and chopped
- ½ teaspoon of dried oregano
- Salt and freshly ground black pepper, to taste
- 4 (5-ounce of) skinless, boneless chicken breasts, butterflied and pounded

Instructions:

1. Preheat your oven to 350 degrees F.
2. Line a baking sheet with parchment paper.
3. In a saucepan, heat the vegetable oil over medium heat and sauté onion and both peppers for about 1 minute.

4. Add the garlic and spinach and cook for about 2-3 minutes or until just wilted.

5. Stir in oregano, salt, and black pepper, and take away the saucepan from heat.

6. Place the chicken mixture into the center of every butterflied chicken breast.

7. Fold each chicken breast over filling to form a touch pocket and secure with toothpicks.

8. Arrange the chicken breasts onto the prepared baking sheet.

9. Bake for about 18-20 minutes.

10. Serve hot.

Chicken & Green Veggies Curry

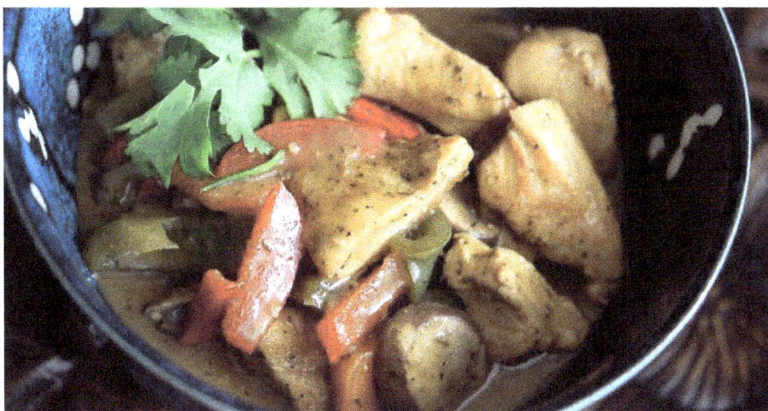

Servings: 4

Preparation Time: 15 minutes

Cooking Time: 30 minutes

Ingredients:

- 1-pound skinless, boneless chicken breasts, cubed
- 1 tablespoon of olive oil
- 2 tablespoons of green curry paste
- 1 cup of unsweetened coconut milk
- 1 cup of low-sodium chicken broth
- 1 cup of asparagus spears, trimmed
- 1 cup of green beans, trimmed
- Salt and ground black pepper, as required

21

- ¼ cup of fresh cilantro leaves, chopped

Instructions:

1. In a skillet, heat oil over medium heat and sauté the curry paste for about 1-2 minutes.
2. Add the chicken and cook for about 8-10 minutes.
3. Add coconut milk and broth and bring to a boil.
4. Reduce the heat low and cook for about 8-10 minutes.
5. Add asparagus, green beans, salt, black pepper and cook for about 4-5 minutes or until desired doneness.
6. Serve hot.

Turkey & Avocado Lettuce Wraps

Servings: 2

Preparation Time: 15 minutes

Cooking Time: 13 minutes

Ingredients:

- 4 ounces of lean ground turkey
- ¼ cup of white onion, minced
- 2 tablespoons of sugar-free tomato sauce
- 1/8 teaspoon of ground cumin
- Freshly ground black pepper, to taste
- 2 teaspoons of extra-virgin olive oil
- 1 cup of tomato, chopped
- ½ cup of avocado, peeled, pitted, and chopped
- 1 tablespoon of fresh cilantro, chopped
- 4 large butternut lettuce leaves

Instructions:

1. In a bowl, add the turkey, onion, pasta sauce, cumin, and black pepper and blend until well combined.
2. In a large skillet, heat the oil over medium heat and cook the turkey mixture for about 8-10 minutes.

3. Add the tomato and stir to mix.
4. Immediately reduce the heat to low and cook for about 2-3 minutes.
5. Remove from the heat and put aside to chill.
6. Arrange the lettuce leaves onto serving plates.
7. Place the turkey mixture over each lettuce leaf evenly and top with avocado pieces.
8. Garnish with cilantro and serve immediately.

Turkey Burgers

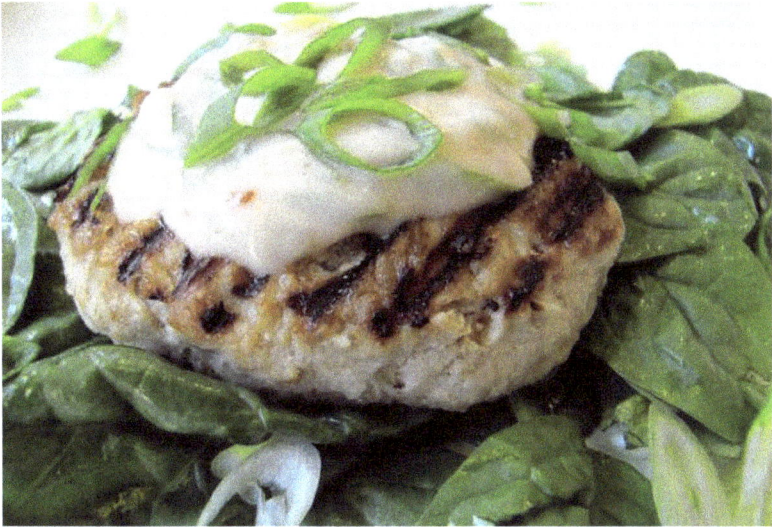

Servings: 2

Preparation Time: 15 minutes

Cooking Time: 6 minutes

Ingredients:

For Burgers:

- 8 ounces of ground turkey
- Salt and ground black pepper, as required
- 1 ounce of part-skim Mozzarella cheese, cubed
- 1 tablespoon of olive oil

For Serving:

- 4 cups of fresh baby spinach
- 1 small cucumber, chopped

Instructions:

1. In a bowl, add the meat, salt, and black pepper and blend until well combined.
2. Make 2 equal-sized patties from the mixture.
3. Place mozzarella cues over each patty, and with your finger, press inside.
4. In a skillet, heat oil over medium heat and cook the patties for about 2-3 minutes per side.
5. Serve immediately alongside the spinach and cucumber.

Turkey, Apple & Veggies Burgers

Servings: 4

Preparation Time: 20 minutes

Cooking Time: 12 minutes

Ingredients:

For Burgers:

- 12 ounces of lean ground turkey
- ½ of apple, peeled, cored, and grated
- ½ of red bell pepper, seeded and chopped finely
- ¼ cup of red onion, minced
- 2 small garlic cloves, minced
- 1 tablespoon of fresh ginger, minced
- 2½ tablespoons of fresh cilantro, chopped
- 2 tablespoons of curry paste
- 1 teaspoon of ground cumin
- 1 teaspoon of olive oil

For Serving:

- 6 cups of fresh baby spinach

Instructions:

1. Preheat the grill to medium heat. Grease the grill grate.
2. For Burgers: in a large bowl, add all the ingredients apart from oil and blend until well combined.
3. Make 4 equal-sized burgers from the mixture.
4. Brush the burgers with vegetable oil evenly.
5. Place the burgers onto the grill and cook for about 5-6 minutes per side.
6. Divide the baby spinach onto serving plates and top each with 1 burger.
7. Serve immediately.

Turkey Stuffed Zucchini

Servings: 8

Preparation Time: 15 minutes

Cooking Time: 31 minutes

Ingredients:

- 4 medium zucchinis
- 1-pound lean ground turkey breast
- ½ cup of white onion, chopped
- ½ pound fresh mushrooms, sliced
- 1 large tomato, chopped
- 1 egg, beaten
- ¾ cup of sugar-free spaghetti sauce
- ¼ cup of seasoned whole wheat bread crumbs
- Freshly ground black pepper, to taste
- 1 cup of low-fat mozzarella cheese, shredded

Instructions:

1. Preheat your oven to 350 degrees F.
2. Cut each zucchini in half lengthwise.
3. With a pointy knife, cut a skinny slice from the rock bottom of every zucchini to permit zucchini to take a seat flat.

4. With a little spoon, scoop out the pulp from each zucchini half, leaving ¼-inch shells.

5. Transfer the zucchini pulp into a large bowl and put it aside.

6. Arrange the zucchini shells into an ungreased microwave-safe baking dish.

7. Cover the baking dish and microwave on High for about 3 minutes.

8. Drain the water from the microwave and put it aside.

9. Heat a large non-stick skillet over medium heat and cook the bottom turkey and onion for about 6-8 minutes or until meat is no longer pink.

10. Drain the grease completely.

11. Remove from the heat.

12. In the bowl of zucchini pulp, add the cooked turkey, mushrooms, tomato, egg, spaghetti sauce, black pepper, and ½ cup of the cheese and blend until well combined.

13. Place about ¼ cup of the turkey mixture into each zucchini shell and sprinkle with the remaining cheese.

14. Bake for about 20 minutes or until the top becomes golden brown.

15. Serve hot.

Turkey Stuffed Acorn Squash

Servings: 4

Preparation Time: 15 minutes

Cooking Time: 50 minutes

Ingredients:

- 2 acorn squash, halved and seeded
- 1-pound lean ground turkey breast
- 1 cup of red onion, chopped
- 1 cup of celery stalk, chopped
- 1 cup of fresh button mushrooms, sliced
- 8 ounces of sugar-free tomato sauce
- 1 teaspoon of dried oregano, crushed
- 1 teaspoon of dried basil, crushed
- Freshly ground black pepper, to taste
- 1 cup of low-fat Cheddar cheese, shredded

Instructions:

1. Preheat your oven to 350 degrees F.
2. In the bottom of a microwave-safe glass baking dish, arrange the squash halves, cut side down.

3. Microwave on High for about 20 minutes or until almost tender.
4. Heat a large non-stick skillet over medium heat and cook the bottom turkey for about 4-5 minutes or until meat is no longer pink.
5. Drain the grease completely.
6. Add the onion and celery and cook for about 3-4 minutes.
7. Stir in the mushrooms and cook for about 2-3 minutes more.
8. Stir in the spaghetti sauce, dried herbs, and black pepper and take away from the heat.
9. Spoon the turkey mixture into each squash half.
10. Cover the baking dish and bake for about 15 minutes.
11. Uncover the baking dish and sprinkle each squash half with cheddar.
12. Bake uncovered for about 3-5 minutes or until the cheese becomes bubbly.
13. Serve hot.

Turkey & Spinach Meatballs

Servings: 4

Preparation Time: 20 minutes

Cooking Time: 15 minutes

Ingredients:

For Meatballs:

- 1-pound lean ground turkey
- 1 cup of frozen chopped spinach, thawed and squeezed
- ½ cup of feta cheese, crumbled
- ½ teaspoon of dried oregano
- Salt and ground black pepper, as required
- 2 tablespoons of olive oil

For Salad:

- 4 cups of lettuce, torn
- 2 large tomatoes, chopped
- 1 cup of onion, sliced
- 2 tablespoons of olive oil
- Salt and ground black pepper, as required

Instructions:

1. For meatballs: place all ingredients apart from oil in a bowl and blend until well combined.
2. Make 12 equal-sized meatballs from the mixture.
3. Heat the vegetable oil in a large non-stick skillet over medium heat and cook the meatballs for about 10-15 minutes or until done completely, flipping occasionally.
4. With a slotted spoon, transfer the meatballs onto a plate.
5. Meanwhile, For Salad: In a large salad bowl, add all ingredients and toss to coat well.
6. Divide meatballs and salad onto serving plates and serve.

Turkey Meatballs Kabobs

Servings: 4

Preparation Time: 15 minutes

Cooking Time: 14 minutes

Ingredients:

- 1 yellow onion, chopped roughly
- ½ cup of lemongrass, chopped roughly
- 2 garlic cloves, chopped roughly
- 1½ pounds of lean ground turkey
- 1 teaspoon of sesame oil
- ½ tablespoons of low-sodium soy sauce
- 1 tablespoon of arrowroot starch
- 1/8 teaspoon of powdered stevia
- Salt and ground black pepper, as required
- 6 cups of fresh baby spinach

Instructions:

1. Preheat the grill to medium-high heat.
2. Grease the grill grate.
3. In a food processor, add the onion, lemongrass, and garlic and pulse until chopped finely.

35

4. Transfer the onion mixture into a large bowl.
5. Add the remaining ingredients apart from spinach and blend until well combined.
6. Make 12 equal-sized balls from the meat mixture.
7. Thread the balls onto the presoaked wooden skewers.
8. Place the skewers onto the grill and cook for about 6-7 minutes per side.
9. Serve hot alongside the spinach.

Turkey with Peas

Servings: 6

Preparation Time: 15 minutes

Cooking Time: 40 minutes

Ingredients:

- 2 tablespoons of extra virgin olive oil
- 1-pound lean ground turkey
- 1 large white onion, chopped finely
- 2 garlic cloves, minced
- ½ tablespoon of fresh ginger, minced
- 1 teaspoon of ground coriander
- 1 teaspoon of ground cumin
- ¼ teaspoon of chili powder
- 2 medium tomatoes, seeded and chopped
- ½ cup of low-sodium chicken broth
- Salt and freshly ground black pepper, to taste
- 2 cups of fresh peas, shelled
- 2 tablespoons of fresh cilantro, chopped

Instructions:

1. In a large skillet, heat the oil over medium heat and cook the turkey for about 4-5 minutes or until browned completely.
2. With a slotted spoon, transfer the turkey into a large bowl.
3. In the same skillet, add the onion and sauté for about 4-6 minutes.
4. Add the garlic, ginger, coriander, cumin, and chili powder and sauté for about 1 minute.
5. Add the tomatoes and cook for about 2-3 minutes, crushing completely with the rear of the spoon.
6. Stir in the cooked turkey, broth, salt, and black pepper and bring to a boil.
7. Reduce the heat to medium-low and simmer, covered for about 8-10 minutes, stirring occasionally.
8. Stir in peas and cook for about 15-20 minutes.
9. Remove from the heat and serve hot with the garnishing of almonds and cilantro leaves.

Turkey & Veggie Casserole

Servings: 6

Preparation Time: 15 minutes

Cooking Time: 50 minutes

Ingredients:

- 2 medium zucchinis, sliced
- 2 medium tomatoes, sliced
- ¾ pound ground turkey
- 1 large yellow onion, chopped
- 2 garlic cloves, minced
- 1 cup of sugar-free tomato sauce
- ½ cup of low-fat cheddar cheese, shredded
- 2 cups of cottage cheese, shredded
- 1 egg yolk
- 1 tablespoon of fresh rosemary, minced
- Salt and ground black pepper, as required

Instructions:

1. Preheat your oven to 500 degrees F.
2. Grease a large roasting pan

3. Arrange zucchini and tomato slices into the prepared roasting pan and spray with some cooking spray.

4. Roast for about 10-12 minutes.

5. Remove from oven and put aside.

6. Now, preheat your oven to 350 degrees F.

7. Meanwhile, heat a nonstick skillet over medium-high heat and cook the turkey for about 4-5 minutes or until browned.

8. Add the onion and garlic and sauté for about 4-5 minutes.

9. Stir in spaghetti sauce and cook for about 2-3 minutes.

10. Remove from the heat and place the turkey mixture into a 13x9-inch shallow baking dish.

11. In a bowl, add the remaining ingredients and blend until well combined.

12. Place the roasted vegetables over the turkey mixture, followed by the cheese mixture evenly.

13. Bake for about 35 minutes.

14. Remove from the oven and put aside for about 5-10 minutes.

15. Cut into equal-sized 8 wedges and serve.

Turkey Chili

Servings: 8

Preparation Time: 15 minutes

Cooking Time: 2¼ hours

Ingredients:

- 2 tablespoons of olive oil
- 1 small yellow onion, chopped
- 1 green bell pepper, seeded and chopped
- 4 garlic cloves, minced
- 1 jalapeño pepper, chopped
- 1 teaspoon of dried thyme, crushed
- 2 tablespoons of red chili powder
- 1 tablespoon of ground cumin
- 2 pounds lean ground turkey
- 2 cups of fresh tomatoes, chopped finely
- 2 ounces of sugar-free tomato paste
- 2 cups of homemade low-sodium chicken broth
- 1 cup of water
- Salt and ground black pepper, as required

Instructions:

1. In a large Dutch oven, heat oil over medium heat and sauté the onion and bell pepper for about 5-7 minutes.
2. Add the garlic, jalapeno, thyme, and spices and sauté for about 1 minute.
3. Add the turkey and cook for about 4-5 minutes.
4. Stir in the tomatoes, ingredient, and cacao powder and cook for about 2 minutes.
5. Add in the broth and water and bring to a boil.
6. Now, reduce the heat to low and simmer, covered for about 2 hours.
7. Add in salt and black pepper and take away from the heat.
8. Serve hot.

Turkey & Veggie Casserole

Servings: 6

Preparation Time: 20 minutes

Cooking Time: 1 hour

Ingredients:

- 2 medium zucchinis, sliced
- 2 medium tomatoes, sliced
- Olive oil cooking spray
- ¾ pound of ground turkey
- 1 large yellow onion, chopped
- 2 garlic cloves, minced
- 1 cup of sugar-free tomato sauce
- ½ cup of low-fat cheddar cheese, shredded
- 2 cups of cottage cheese, shredded
- 1 egg yolk
- 1 tablespoon of fresh rosemary, minced
- Salt and ground black pepper, as required

Instructions:

1. Preheat your oven to 500 degrees F.
2. Grease a large roasting pan.

3. Arrange zucchini and tomato slices into the prepared roasting pan and spray with some cooking spray.
4. Roast for about 10-12 minutes.
5. Remove from oven and put aside.
6. Now, preheat your oven to 350 degrees F.
7. Meanwhile, heat a non-stick skillet over medium-high heat and cook the turkey for about 4-5 minutes or until brown.
8. Add the onion and garlic and sauté for about 4-5 minutes.
9. Stir in spaghetti sauce and cook for about 2-3 minutes.
10. Remove from the heat and place the turkey mixture into a 13x9-inch shallow baking dish.
11. In a bowl, add the remaining ingredients and blend until well combined.
12. Place the roasted vegetables over the turkey mixture, followed by the cheese mixture evenly.
13. Bake for about 35 minutes.
14. Remove from the oven and put aside for about 5-10 minutes.
15. Divide into desired sized pieces and serve.

Beef Lettuce Wraps

Servings: 2

Preparation Time: 15 minutes

Cooking Time: 13 minutes

Ingredients:

- 2 tablespoons of white onion, chopped
- 5 ounces of lean ground beef
- 2 tablespoons of light thousand island dressing
- 1/8 teaspoon of white vinegar
- 1/8 teaspoon of onion powder
- 4 lettuce leaves
- 2 tablespoons of low-fat cheddar cheese, shredded
- 1 small cucumber, julienned

Instructions:

1. Heat a little, lightly greased skillet over medium-high heat, and sauté the onion for about 2-3 minutes.
2. Add the meat and cook for about 8-10 minutes or until cooked through.
3. Remove from the heat and put aside.

4. In a bowl, add the dressing, vinegar, and onion powder and blend well.
5. Arrange the lettuce leaves onto serving plates.
6. Place beef mixture over each lettuce leaf, followed by the cheese and cucumber.
7. Drizzle with sauce and serve.

Simple Beef Burgers

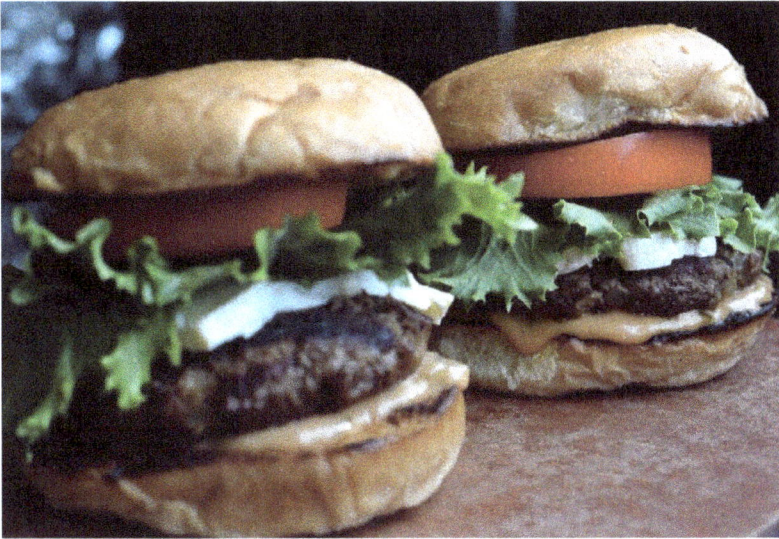

Servings: 4

Preparation Time: 15 minutes

Cooking Time: 10 minutes

Ingredients:

- 1-pound ground beef
- 1 large egg, lightly beaten
- ½ cup of seasoned breadcrumbs
- Salt and ground black pepper, as required
- 1 tablespoon of olive oil

- 6 cups of fresh spinach, torn
- 1 large tomato, chopped

Instructions:

1. Preheat the grill to medium heat.
2. Grease the grill grate.
3. In a large bowl, add the meat, egg, breadcrumbs, salt, black pepper and blend until well combined.
4. Make 4 (½-inch thick) patties from the mixture.
5. With your thumb, press a shallow indentation in the center of every patty.
6. Brush each side of every patty with oil.
7. Place the burgers onto the grill and cook, covered for about 4-5 minutes per side.
8. Serve alongside the spinach and tomato.

Beef & Spinach Burgers

Servings: 4

Preparation Time: 15 minutes

Cooking Time: 12 minutes

Ingredients:

For Burgers:

- 1-pound ground beef
- 1 cup of fresh baby spinach leaves, chopped
- ½ of small yellow onion, chopped
- ¼ cup of sun-dried tomatoes, chopped
- 1 egg, beaten
- ¼ cup of feta cheese, crumbled
- Salt and ground black pepper, as required
- 2 tablespoons of olive oil

For Serving:

- 3 cups of fresh spinach, torn
- 3 cups of lettuce, torn
- 2 tomatoes, sliced

Instructions:

1. For Burgers: in a large bowl, add all ingredients apart from oil and blend until well combined.
2. Make 4 equal-sized patties from the mixture.
3. In a skillet, heat the oil over medium-high heat and cook the patties for about 5-6 minutes per side or until desired doneness.
4. Divide the lettuce, spinach, and tomato slices and onto serving plates.
5. Top each with 1 burger and serve.

Spicy Beef Burgers

Servings: 4

Preparation Time: 20 minutes

Cooking Time: 10 minutes

Ingredients:

For Burgers

- 1-pound lean ground beef
- ¼ cup of fresh parsley, chopped
- ¼ cup of fresh parsley, chopped
- ¼ cup of fresh cilantro, chopped
- 1 tablespoon of fresh ginger, chopped
- 1 teaspoon of ground cumin
- 1 teaspoon of ground coriander
- ½ teaspoon of ground cinnamon
- Salt and ground black pepper, as required
- For Salad:
- 6 cup of fresh baby arugula
- 2 cups of cherry tomatoes, quartered
- 1 tablespoon of fresh lemon juice
- 1 tablespoon of extra-virgin olive oil

Instructions:

1. In a bowl, add the meat, ¼ cup of parsley, cilantro, ginger, spices, salt, and black pepper, and blend until well combined.
2. Make 4 equal-sized patties from the mixture.
3. Heat a greased grill pan over medium-high heat and cook the patties for about 3 minutes per side or until desired doneness.
4. Meanwhile, in a bowl, add arugula, tomatoes, juice, oil, and toss to coat well.
5. Divide the salad onto serving plates and top each with 1 patty.
6. Serve immediately.

Spiced Beef Meatballs

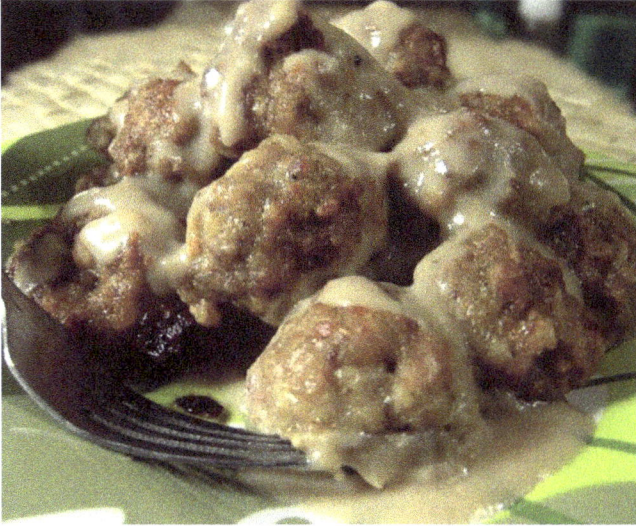

Servings: 4

Preparation Time: 15 minutes

Cooking Time: 20 minutes

Ingredients:

- 1-pound of ground beef
- 1 tablespoon of olive oil
- 1 teaspoon of dehydrated onion flakes, crushed
- ½ teaspoon of granulated garlic
- ½ teaspoon of ground cumin

- ½ teaspoon of red pepper flakes, crushed
- Salt, as required
- 6 cups of fresh baby spinach
- 1 cup of tomato, chopped

Instructions:

1. Preheat the oven to 400 degrees F.
2. Line a bigger baking sheet with parchment paper.
3. In a bowl, place all the ingredients and with your hands, mix until well combined.
4. Shape the mixture into desired and equal-sized balls.
5. Arrange meatballs into the prepared baking sheet in a single layer and Bake for about 15-20 minutes or until done completely.
6. Serve hot alongside spinach and tomato.

Beef & Veggie Meatballs

Servings: 6

Preparation Time: 15 minutes

Cooking Time: 30 minutes

Ingredients:

For Meatballs:

- ½ cup of carrot, peeled and grated
- ½ cup of zucchini, grated
- ½ cup of yellow squash, grated
- Salt, as required
- 1-pound lean ground beef
- 1 egg, beaten
- ¼ of a small onion, chopped finely
- 1 garlic clove, minced
- 2 tablespoons of mixed fresh herbs (parsley, basil, cilantro, chopped final

For Serving:

- 6 cups of fresh baby spinach
- 3 large tomatoes, sliced

Instructions:

1. Preheat your oven to 400 degrees F.
2. Line a large baking sheet with parchment paper.
3. In a large colander, place the carrot, zucchini and yellow squash and sprinkle with 2 pinches of salt. Put aside for at least 10 minutes.
4. Transfer the veggies over a towel and squeeze out all the moisture
5. In a large bowl, add squeezed vegetables, beef, egg, onion, garlic, herbs, salt, and blend until well combined.
6. Shape the mixture into equal-sized balls.
7. Arrange the meatballs onto the prepared baking sheet in a single layer.
8. Bake for about 25-30 minutes or until done completely.
9. Divide the spinach and tomato slices onto serving plates.
10. Top each plate with meatballs and serve.

Spicy Beef Koftas

Servings: 6

Preparation Time: 15 minutes

Cooking Time: 10 minutes

Ingredients:

- 1-pound ground beef
- 2 tablespoons of low-fat plain Greek yoghurt
- 2 tablespoons of yellow onion, grated
- 2 teaspoons of garlic, minced
- 2 tablespoons of fresh cilantro, minced
- 1 teaspoon of ground coriander
- 1 teaspoon of ground cumin
- 1 teaspoon of ground turmeric
- Salt and ground black pepper, as required
- 1 tablespoon of olive oil
- 8 cups of fresh salad greens

Instructions:

1. In a large bowl, add all the ingredients apart from greens and blend until well combined.
2. Make 12 equal-sized oblong patties from the mixture.

3. In a large non-stick skillet, heat the oil over medium-high heat and cook the patties for about 10 minutes or until browned from each side, flipping occasionally.

4. Meanwhile, for sauce: In a bowl, add all the ingredients and blend until well combined.

5. Serve the Koftas with the yoghurt sauce.

Beef Kabobs

Servings: 6

Preparation Time: 15 minutes

Cooking Time: 8 minutes

Ingredients:

- 3 garlic cloves, minced
- 1 tablespoon of fresh lemon zest, grated
- 2 teaspoons of fresh rosemary, minced
- 2 teaspoons of fresh parsley, minced
- 2 teaspoons of fresh oregano, minced
- 2 teaspoons of fresh thyme, minced
- 4 tablespoons of olive oil
- 2 tablespoons of fresh lemon juice
- Salt and ground black pepper, as required
- 2 pounds beef sirloin, cut into cubes
- 8 cups of fresh baby greens

Instructions:

1. In a bowl, add all the ingredients except the meat and greens and blend well.
2. Add the meat and coat with the herb mixture generously.

3. Refrigerate to marinate for at least 20-30 minutes.

4. Preheat the grill to medium-high heat. Grease the grill grate.

5. Remove the meat cubes from the marinade and thread onto metal skewers.

6. Place the skewers onto the grill and cook for about 6-8 minutes, flipping after every 2 minutes.

7. Remove from the grill and place onto a platter for about 5 minutes before serving.

8. Serve alongside the greens.

Garlicky Beef Tenderloin

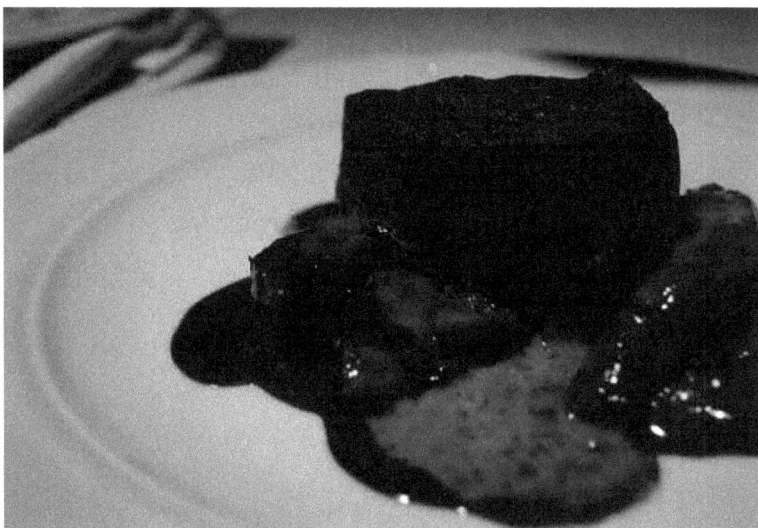

Servings: 19

Preparation Time: 10 minutes

Cooking Time: 50 minutes

Ingredients:

- 1 (3-pound) centre-cut beef tenderloin roast
- 4 garlic cloves, minced
- 1 tablespoon of fresh rosemary, minced
- Salt and ground black pepper, to taste
- 1 tablespoon of olive oil

- 15 cups of fresh spinach

Instructions:

1. Preheat your oven to 425 degrees F.
2. Grease a large shallow roasting pan.
3. Place the roast into the prepared roasting pan.
4. Rub the roast with garlic, rosemary, salt, and black pepper, and drizzle with oil.
5. Roast the meat for about 45-50 minutes.
6. Remove from oven and place the roast onto a chopping board for about 10 minutes.
7. With a knife, cut tenderloin into desired-sized slices and serve alongside the spinach.

Simple Steak

Servings: 4

Preparation Time: 10 minutes

Cooking Time: 10 minutes

Ingredients:

- 1 tablespoon of olive oil
- 4 (6-ounce of) flank steaks
- Salt and ground black pepper, to taste
- 6 cups of fresh salad greens

Instructions:

1. In a wok, heat the oil over medium-high heat and cook steaks with salt and black pepper for about 3-5 minutes per side.

2. Transfer the steaks onto serving plates and serve alongside the greens.

Rosemary Steak

Servings: 6

Preparation Time: 15 minutes

Cooking Time: 15 minutes

Ingredients:

- 3 garlic cloves, minced
- 2 tablespoons of fresh rosemary, chopped
- Salt and ground black pepper, as required
- 2 pounds flank steak, trimmed
- 8 cups of fresh baby kale

Instructions:

1. Preheat the grill to medium-high heat.
2. Grease the grill grate.
3. In a large bowl, add all the ingredients except the steak and kale mix until well combined.
4. Add the steak and coat with the mixture generously.
5. Put aside for about 10 minutes.
6. Place the steak onto the grill and cook for about 12-15 minutes, flipping after every 3-4 minutes.

7. Remove from the grill and place the steak onto a chopping board for about 5 minutes.
8. Meanwhile, for sauce: in a bowl, add all the ingredients and blend well.
9. With a pointy knife, cut the steak into desired sized slices.
10. Serve the steak slices alongside the kale.

Spiced Flank Steak

Servings: 5

Preparation Time: 10 minutes

Cooking Time: 20 minutes

Ingredients:

- ½ teaspoon of dried thyme, crushed
- ½ teaspoon of dried oregano, crushed
- 1 teaspoon of red chili powder
- ½ teaspoon of ground cumin
- ¼ teaspoon of garlic powder
- Salt and ground black pepper, to taste
- 1½ pounds flank steak, trimmed
- 6 cups of salad greens

Instructions:

1. In a large bowl, add the dried herbs and spices and blend well.
2. Add the steaks and rub with mixture generously.
3. Put aside for about 15-20 minutes.
4. Preheat the grill to medium heat. Grease the grill grate.

5. Place the steak onto the grill over medium coals and cook for about 18–20 minutes, flipping once halfway through.
6. Remove the steak from grill and place onto a chopping board for about 10 minutes before slicing.

7. With a knife, cut the steak into desired sized slices and serve alongside the greens.

Simple Flank Steak

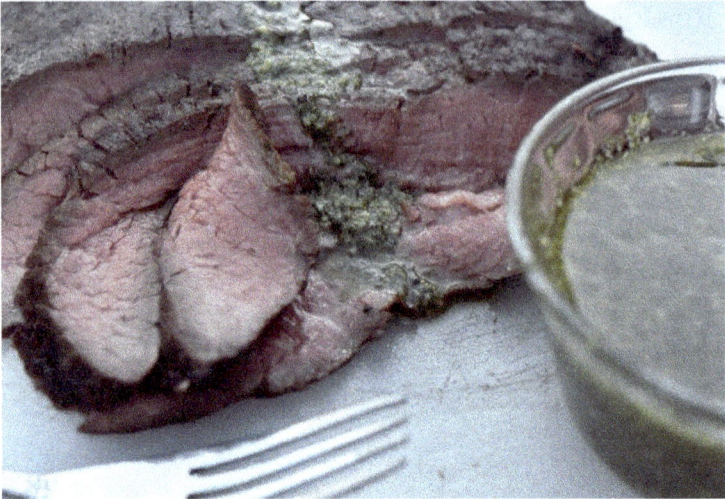

Servings: 4

Preparation Time: 10 minutes

Cooking Time: 8 minutes

Ingredients:

For Steak:

- 2 tablespoons of extra-virgin olive oil
- 4 (6-ounce of) flank steaks
- Salt and ground black pepper, to taste

For Salad:

- 6 cups of fresh baby arugula
- 3 tablespoons of extra-virgin olive oil
- 2 tablespoons of balsamic vinegar
- Salt and ground black pepper, to taste

Instructions:

1. In a sauté pan, heat the oil over medium-high heat and cook the steaks with salt and black pepper for about 3-4 minutes per side.
2. Meanwhile, For Salad: in a salad bowl, place all ingredients and toss to coat well.
3. Divide the arugula onto serving plates and top each with 1 steak.
4. Serve immediately.

Steak with Green Beans

Servings: 2

Preparation Time: 15 minutes

Cooking Time: 10 minutes

Ingredients:

For Steak:

- 2 (5-ounce of) sirloin steaks, trimmed
- Salt and ground black pepper, as required
- 1 tablespoon of extra-virgin olive oil
- 1 garlic clove, minced

For Green Beans:

- ½ pound fresh green beans
- ½ tablespoon of olive oil
- ½ tablespoon of fresh lemon juice

Instructions:

1. For steak: Season the steaks with salt and black pepper evenly.
2. In a forged iron sauté pan, heat the vegetable oil over high heat and sauté garlic for about 15-20 seconds.

3. Add the steaks and cook for about 3 minutes per side.
4. Flip the steaks and cook for about 3-4 minutes or until the desired doneness, flipping once.
5. Meanwhile, for green beans: in a pan of boiling water, arrange a steamer basket.
6. Place the green beans in a steamer basket and steam covered for about 4-5 minutes.
7. Carefully transfer the beans into a bowl.
8. Add vegetable oil and juice and toss to coat well.
9. Divide green beans onto serving plates.
10. Top each with 1 steak and serve.

Veggie & Feta Stuffed Steak

Servings: 6

Preparation Time: 15 minutes

Cooking Time: 35 minutes

Ingredients:

- 12 tablespoons of dried oregano leaves
- 1/3 cup of fresh lemon juice
- 2 tablespoons of olive oil
- 1 (2-pound) beef flank steak, pounded into ½-inch thickness.
- 1/3 cup of olive tapenade
- 1 cup of frozen chopped spinach, thawed and squeezed
- ¼ cup of feta cheese, crumbled
- 4 cups of fresh cherry tomatoes
- Salt, as required

Instructions:

1. In a large baking dish, add the oregano, juice and oil and blend well.
2. Add the steak and coat with the marinade generously.

3. Refrigerate to marinate for about 4 hours, flipping occasionally.
4. Preheat the oven to 425 degrees F.
5. Line a shallow baking dish with parchment paper.
6. Remove the steak from baking dish, reserving the remaining marinade in a bowl.
7. Cover the bowl of marinade and refrigerate.
8. Arrange the steak onto a chopping board.
9. Place the tapenade onto the steak evenly and top with the spinach, followed by the feta cheese.
1. 10 Carefully roll the steak tightly to make a log.
10. With 6 kitchen string pieces, tie the log at 6 places.
11. Carefully cut the log between strings into 6 equal pieces, leaving string in place.
12. In a bowl, add the reserved marinade, tomatoes and salt and toss to coat.
13. Arrange the log pieces onto the prepared baking dish, cut-side up.
14. Now, arrange the tomatoes around the pinwheels evenly.
15. Bake for about 25-35 minutes.
16. Remove from the oven and put aside for about 5 minutes before serving.

Beef & Broccoli Bowl

Serving: 1

Preparation Time: 15 minutes

Cooking Time: 12 minutes

Ingredients:

- 4 ounces of lean ground beef
- 1 cup of broccoli, cut into bite-sized pieces
- 2 tablespoons of low-sodium chicken broth
- ¼ cup of tomatoes, chopped
- ¼ teaspoon of onion powder
- ¼ teaspoon of garlic powder
- Pinch of red pepper flakes
- Salt, to taste
- 1 ounce of low-fat cheddar cheese

Instructions:

1. Heat a lightly greased skillet over medium heat and cook the meat for about 8-10 minutes or until browned completely.
2. Meanwhile, in a microwave-safe bowl, place the broccoli and broth.

3. With a plastic wrap, cover the bowl and microwave for about 4 minutes.
4. Remove from the microwave and put aside.
5. Drain the grease from skillet.
6. Add the tomatoes, garlic powder, onion powder, red pepper flakes and salt and stir to mix well.
7. Add the broccoli and toss to coat well.
8. Remove from the heat and transfer the meat mixture into a serving bowl.
9. Top with cheddar and serve.

Beef Taco Bowl

Servings: 4

Preparation Time: 15 minutes

Cooking Time: 15 minutes

Ingredients:

- 1 teaspoon of red chili powder
- 1 teaspoon of ground cumin
- Salt and freshly ground black pepper, to taste
- 1-pound flank steak, trimmed
- 2 scallions
- 1 lime, cut in half
- 8 cup of lettuce, torn
- 1 red bell pepper, seeded and sliced
- 1 cup of tomato, chopped
- ½ cup of fresh cilantro, chopped
- ¼ cup of light sour cream

Instructions:

1. Preheat the grill to medium-high heat. Grease the grill grate.

2. In a small bowl, mix together the spices, salt and black pepper.
3. Rub the steak with spice mixture generously.
4. Place the steak onto the grill and cook for about 4-6 minutes per side or until desired doneness.
5. Remove from the grill and place the steak onto a chopping board for about 5 minutes.
6. Now, place the scallions onto the grill and cook for about 1 minute per side.
7. Place the lime halves onto the grill, cut-side down and cook for about 1 minute.
8. Remove the scallions and lime halves from the grill and place onto a plate.
9. Chop the scallions roughly.
10. With a pointy knife, cut the steak into thin slices.
11. In a bowl, place the meat slices and chopped scallions.
12. Squeeze the lime halves over steak mixture and toss to coat well.
13. Divide lettuce into serving bowls and top each with bell pepper, followed by tomato, cilantro and beef mixture.
14. Top each bowl with soured cream and serve.

Veggie Stuffed Steak

Servings: 4

Preparation Time: 15 minutes

Cooking Time: 35 minutes

Ingredients:

- 1 (1½-pound) flank steak
- Salt and freshly ground black pepper, to taste
- 1 tablespoon of olive oil
- 2 small garlic cloves, minced
- 6 ounces of fresh spinach, chopped finely
- 1 medium green bell pepper, seeded and chopped
- 1 medium tomato, chopped finely

Instructions:

1. Preheat your oven to 425 degrees F. Grease a large baking dish.
2. Place beefsteak onto a flat surface.
3. Hold a pointy knife parallel to figure surface, slice the steak horizontally, without cutting all the way through, that you simply can open sort of a book.

4. With a meat mallet, flatten the steak to a good thickness. Sprinkle the steak with salt and black pepper evenly.
5. In a skillet, heat oil over medium heat and sauté garlic for about 1 minute.
6. Add spinach, with salt and black pepper and cook for about 2 minutes.
7. Stir in bell pepper and tomato and immediately remove from heat.
8. Transfer the spinach into a bowl and put aside to chill slightly.
9. Place the filling on the top of steak evenly.
10. Roll up the steak to seal the filling.
11. With cotton twine, tie the steak.
12. Place the steak roll into the prepared baking dish.
1. 13 Roast for about 30-35 minutes.
13. Remove from oven and let it cool slightly.
14. With a pointy knife, cut the roll into desired sized slices and serve.

Steak with Broccoli

Servings: 4

Preparation Time: 15 minutes

Cooking Time: 20 minutes

Ingredients:

- 16 ounces of sirloin steak, trimmed and cut into thin strips
- Salt and freshly ground black pepper, to taste
- 2 tablespoons of olive oil, divided
- 2 garlic cloves, minced
- 1 Serrano pepper, seeded and chopped finely
- 2 cups of broccoli florets
- 2 tablespoons of low-sodium soy sauce
- 2 tablespoons of fresh lime juice

Instructions:

1. Season the steak slices with black pepper.
2. Heat 1 tablespoon of oil in a large skillet over medium heat and cook the steak slices for about 6-8 minutes or until browned from all sides.
3. With a slotted spoon, transfer the steak slices onto a plate.

4. Heat remaining oil in the same skillet over medium heat and sauté the garlic and Serrano pepper for about 1 minute.
5. Add the broccoli and fry for about 2-3 minutes.
6. Stir in the cooked steak slices, soy and juice and cook for about 3-4 minutes.
7. Serve hot.

Beef with Mushrooms

Servings: 4

Preparation Time: 15 minutes

Cooking Time: 15 minutes

Ingredients:

For Beef:

- 4 (6-ounce of) beef tenderloin fillets
- Salt and freshly ground black pepper, to taste
- 2 tablespoons of olive oil, divided
- 1 teaspoon of garlic, smashed
- 1 tablespoon of fresh thyme, chopped

For Mushrooms:

- 2 tablespoons of olive oil
- 1-pound fresh mushrooms, sliced
- 2 teaspoons of garlic, smashed
- Salt and freshly ground black pepper, to taste

Instructions:

1. For beef: season the meat fillets with salt and black pepper evenly and put aside.

2. In a cast-iron skillet, heat the oil over medium heat and sauté the garlic and thyme for about 1 minute.
3. Add the fillets and cook for about 5-7 minutes per side.
4. Meanwhile, for mushrooms: in another cast-iron skillet, heat the oil over medium heat and cook the mushrooms, garlic, salt, and black pepper for about 7-8 minutes, stirring frequently.
5. Divide the fillets onto serving plates.
6. Top with mushroom mixture and serve.

Steak with Carrot & Kale

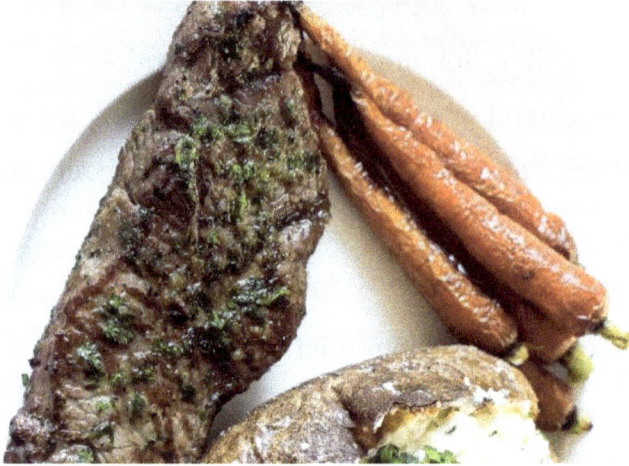

Servings: 4

Preparation Time: 15 minutes

Cooking Time: 12 minutes

Ingredients:

- 2 tablespoons of olive oil
- 4 garlic cloves, minced
- 1-pound beef sirloin steak, cut into bite-sized pieces
- Freshly ground black pepper, to taste
- 1½ cups of carrots, peeled and cut into matchsticks
- 1½ cups of fresh kale, tough ribs removed and chopped

- 3 tablespoons of low-sodium soy sauce

Instructions:

1. In a skillet, heat the oil over medium heat and sauté the garlic for about 1 minute.
2. Add the meat and black pepper and stir to mix.
3. Increase the heat to medium-high and cook for about 3-4 minutes or until browned from all sides.
4. Add the carrot, kale and soy and cook for about 4-5 minutes.
5. Stir in the black pepper and take away from the heat.
6. Serve hot.

Ground Beef with Veggies

Servings: 4

Preparation Time: 15 minutes

Cooking Time: 25 minutes

Ingredients:

- 1-pound lean ground beef
- 2 tablespoons of extra-virgin olive oil
- 2 garlic cloves, minced
- ½ of yellow onion, chopped
- 2 cups of fresh mushrooms, sliced
- 1 cup of fresh kale, tough ribs removed and chopped
- ¼ cup of low-sodium beef broth
- 2 tablespoons of balsamic vinegar
- 2 tablespoons of fresh parsley, chopped

Instructions:

1. Heat a large non-stick skillet over medium-high heat and cook the ground beef for about 8-10 minutes, ending the chunks with a wooden spoon.
2. With a slotted spoon, transfer the meat into a bowl.

3. In the same skillet, add the onion and garlic for about 3 minutes.
4. Add the mushrooms and cook for about 5-minutes.
5. Add the cooked beef, kale, broth and vinegar and bring to a boil.
6. Reduce the heat to medium-low and simmer for about 3 minutes.
7. Stir in parsley and serve immediately.

Beef Chili

Servings: 8

Preparation Time: 15 minutes

Cooking Time: 1¾ hours

Ingredients:

- 2 tablespoons of olive oil
- 3 pounds ground beef
- 1 cup of yellow onion, chopped finely
- ½ cup of celery, chopped finely
- ½ cup of green bell pepper, seeded and chopped finely
- ½ cup of red bell pepper, seeded and chopped finely
- 1 (15-ounce of) can crushed tomatoes with juice
- 1½ cups of tomato juice
- 1½ teaspoons of Worcestershire sauce
- ½ teaspoon of dried oregano
- 3 tablespoons of red chili powder
- 1 teaspoon of ground cumin
- 1 teaspoon of garlic powder
- 1 teaspoon of salt
- ½ teaspoon of ground black pepper

Instructions:

1. In a large pan, heat the oil over medium-high heat and cook the meat for about 8-10 minutes or until browned.

2. Drain the grease from pan, leaving about 2 tablespoons inside.

3. In the pan, add the onions, celery and bell peppers over medium-high heat and cook for about 5 minutes, stirring frequently.

4. Add the tomatoes, tomato juice, Worcester sauce, oregano, spices, and stir to mix.

5. Reduce the heat to low and simmer, covered for about 1-1½ hours, stirring occasionally.

6. Serve hot.

Beef Stuffed Bell Peppers

Servings: 5

Preparation Time: 20 minutes

Cooking Time: 40 minutes

Ingredients:

- 5 large bell peppers, tops and seeds removed
- 1 tablespoon of olive oil
- ½ of large onion, chopped
- ½ teaspoon of dried oregano
- ½ teaspoon of dried thyme
- Salt and ground black pepper, as required
- 1-pound ground beef
- 1 large zucchini, chopped
- 3 tablespoons of homemade tomato paste

Instructions:

1. Preheat your oven to 350 degrees F.
2. Grease a little baking dish.
3. In a large pan of the boiling water, place the bell peppers and cook for about 4-5 minutes.

4. Remove from the water and place onto a paper towel, cut side down.
5. Meanwhile, in a large nonstick wok, heat the vegetable oil over medium heat and sauté onion for about 3-4 minutes.
6. Add the ground beef, oregano, salt, and pepper and cook for about 8-10 minutes.
7. Add the zucchini and cook for about 2-3 minutes.
8. Remove from the heat and drain any juices from the meat mixture.
9. Add the ingredient and stir to mix.
10. Arrange the bell peppers into the prepared baking dish, cut side upward.
11. Stuff the bell peppers with the meat mixture evenly.
12. Bake for about 15 minutes.
13. Serve warm.

Garlicky Pork Tenderloin

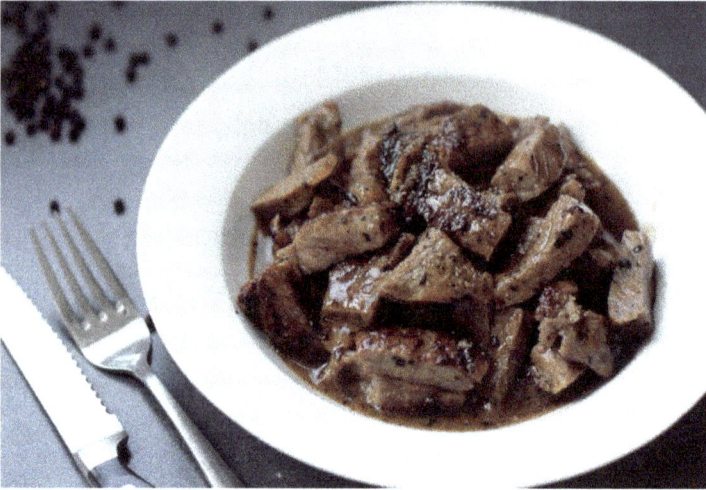

Servings: 6

Preparation Time: 10 minutes

Cooking Time: 38 minutes

Ingredients:

- 3 medium garlic cloves, minced
- 3 teaspoons of dried rosemary, crushed
- ½ teaspoon of cayenne pepper
- Salt and ground black pepper, as required
- 2 pounds pork tenderloin
- 10 cups of fresh baby spinach

Instructions:

1. Preheat the oven to 400 degrees F.

2. Grease a roasting pan.

3. In a bowl, mix together all the ingredients apart from pork and spinach.

4. Rub the pork with garlic mixture evenly.

5. Place the pork into prepared roasting pan.

6. Roast for about 25 minutes or until desired doneness.

7. Remove the roasting pan from oven and place the tenderloin onto a chopping board for about 10-15 minutes.

8. With a pointy knife, cut the tenderloin into desired size slices and serve alongside spinach.

Pork Stuffed Avocado

Servings: 8

Preparation Time: 15 minutes

Cooking Time: 10 minutes

Ingredients:

- 4 ripe avocados, halved and pitted
- 3 tablespoons of fresh lime juice
- 1 tablespoon of olive oil
- 1 medium onion, chopped
- 1-pound ground pork
- 1 packet taco seasoning
- Salt and ground black pepper, as required
- 2/3 cup of low-fat Mexican cheese, shredded
- ½ cup of lettuce, shredded
- ½ cup of cherry tomatoes, quartered

Instructions:

1. Carefully remove abut about 2-3 tablespoons of flesh from each avocado half.
2. Chop the avocado flesh and reserve it.

3. Arrange the avocado halves onto a tray and drizzle each with lime juice.
4. In a medium skillet, heat oil over medium heat and sauté the onion for about 5 minutes.
5. Add the ground pork, taco seasoning, salt and black pepper and cook for about 8-10 minutes, ending the meat with a wooden spoon.
6. Remove from the heat and drain the grease from the skillet.
7. Stuff each avocado half with pork and top with reserved avocado, cheese, lettuce and tomato.
8. Serve immediately.

Pork Burgers

Servings: 4

Preparation Time: 15 minutes

Cooking Time: 6 minutes

Ingredients:

For Patties:

- 1-pound lean ground pork
- ¼ cup of fresh parsley, chopped
- ¼ cup of fresh cilantro, chopped
- 1 tablespoon of fresh ginger, chopped
- 1 teaspoon of ground cumin
- 1 teaspoon of ground coriander
- ½ teaspoon of ground cinnamon
- Salt and ground black pepper, as required

For Salad:

- 6 cups of fresh baby arugula
- 2 cups of cherry tomatoes, quartered
- 1 tablespoon of fresh lemon juice
- 1 tablespoon of extra-virgin olive oil

Instructions:

1. In a bowl, add the pork, parsley, cilantro, ginger, spices, salt and black pepper and blend until well combined.
2. Make 4 equal-sized patties from the mixture.
3. Heat a greased grill pan over medium-high heat and cook the patties for about 3 minutes per side or until desired doneness.
4. Meanwhile, in a bowl, add arugula, tomatoes, juice, oil, and toss to coat well.
5. Divide the salad onto serving plates and top each with 1 patty.
6. Serve immediately.

Pork & Veggie Burgers

Servings: 4

Preparation Time: 15 minutes

Cooking Time: 16 minutes

Ingredients:

For Patties:

- 1-pound ground pork
- 1 carrot, peeled and chopped finely
- 1 medium raw beetroot, trimmed, peeled and chopped finely
- 1 small onion, chopped finely
- 2 Serrano peppers, seeded and chopped
- 1 tablespoon of fresh cilantro, chopped finely
- Salt and ground black pepper, as required
- 3 tablespoons of olive oil

For Burgers:

- 1 large onion, sliced
- 2 large tomatoes, sliced
- 4 lettuce leaves

Instructions:

1. For patties: in a large bowl, add all ingredients apart from oil and blend until well combined.
2. Make equal-sized 8 patties from the mixture.
3. In a large non-stick sauté pan, heat the vegetable oil over medium heat and cook the patties in 2 batches for about 3-4 minutes per side or until golden brown.
4. Arrange the bun bottoms onto serving plates.
5. Plce1 patty over each bun, followed by the onion, tomato and lettuce.
6. Cover each with top of the bun and serve.

Rosemary Pork Tenderloin

Servings: 3

Preparation Time: 10 minutes

Cooking Time: 22 minutes

Ingredients:

- 1 teaspoon of fresh rosemary, minced
- 1 garlic clove, minced
- 1 tablespoon of fresh lemon juice
- 1 tablespoon of olive oil
- 1 teaspoon of Dijon mustard
- 1 teaspoon of powdered Erythritol
- Salt and ground black pepper, to taste
- 1-pound pork tenderloin
- 5 cups of fresh baby kale

Instructions:

1. Preheat your oven to 400 degrees F.
2. Grease a large rimmed baking sheet.
3. In a bowl, place all ingredients except the tenderloin and cheese and beat until well combined.
4. Add tenderloin and coat with the mixture generously.

5. Arrange the tenderloin onto the prepared baking sheet.

6. Bake for about 20-22 minutes.

7. Remove baking sheet from the oven and place the tenderloin onto a chopping board for about 5 minutes.

8. With a pointy knife, cut the tenderloin into ¾-inch-thick slices and serve alongside the kale.

Pork with Veggies

Servings: 4

Preparation Time: 15 minutes

Cooking Time: 15 minutes

Ingredients:

- 1-pound pork loin, cut into thin strips
- 2 tablespoons of olive oil, divided
- 1 teaspoon of garlic, minced
- 1 teaspoon of fresh ginger, minced
- 2 tablespoons of low-sodium soy sauce
- 1 tablespoon of fresh lemon juice
- 1 tablespoon of Erythritol
- 1 teaspoon of arrowroot starch
- 10 ounces of broccoli florets
- 1 carrot, peeled and sliced
- 1 large red bell pepper, seeded and cut into strips
- 2 scallions, cut into 2-inch pieces

Instructions:

1. In a bowl, mix well pork strips, ½ tablespoon of olive oil, garlic, and ginger.

2. For sauce; add the soy sauce, lemon juice, Erythritol, and arrowroot starch in a small bowl and blend well.
3. Heat the remaining vegetable oil in a large nonstick skillet over high heat and sear the pork strips for about 3-4 minutes or until cooked through.
4. With a slotted spoon, transfer the pork into a bowl.
5. In the same skillet, add the carrot and cook for about 2-3 minutes.
6. Add the broccoli, bell pepper, and scallion and cook, covered for about 1-2 minutes.
7. Stir the cooked pork and sauce, and fry and cook for about 3-5 minutes or until the desired doneness, stirring occasionally.
8. Remove from the heat and serve.

Salmon Lettuce Wraps

Servings: 2

Preparation Time: 10 minutes

Ingredients:

- ¼ cup of low-fat mozzarella cheese, cubed
- ¼ cup of tomato, chopped
- 2 tablespoons of fresh dill, chopped
- 1 teaspoon of fresh lemon juice
- Salt, as required
- 4 lettuce leaves
- 1/3 pound cooked salmon, chopped

Instructions:

1. In a small bowl, combine mozzarella, tomato, dill, lemon juice, and salt until well combined.
2. Arrange the lettuce leaves onto serving plates.
3. Divide the salmon and tomato mixture over each lettuce leaf and serve immediately.

Tuna Burgers

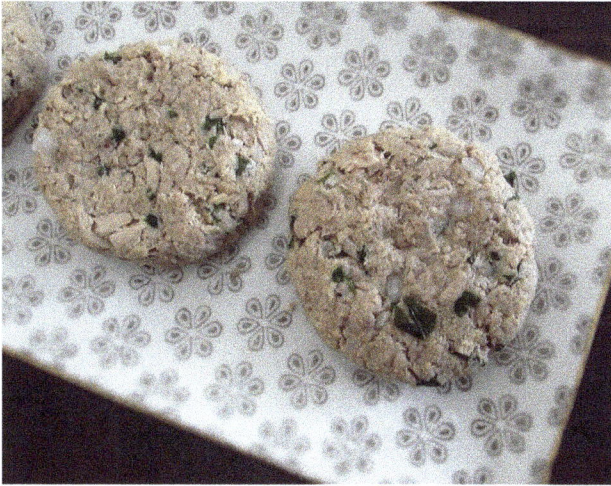

Servings: 2

Preparation Time: 15 minutes

Cooking Time: 6 minutes

Ingredients:

- 1 (15-ounce of) can water-packed tuna, drained
- ½ celery stalk, chopped
- 2 tablespoons of fresh parsley, chopped
- 1 teaspoon of fresh dill, chopped
- 2 tablespoon of walnuts, chopped
- 2 tablespoon of mayonnaise

- 1 egg, beaten
- 1 tablespoon of butter
- 3 cups of lettuce

Instructions:

1. For Burgers: add all ingredients except the butter and lettuce in a bowl and blend until well combined.
2. Make 2 equal-sized patties from the mixture.
3. In a frying pan, melt butter over medium heat and cook the patties for about 2-3 minutes.
4. Carefully flip the side and cook for about 2-3 minutes.
5. Divide the lettuce onto serving plates.
6. Top each plate with 1 burger and serve.

Spicy Salmon

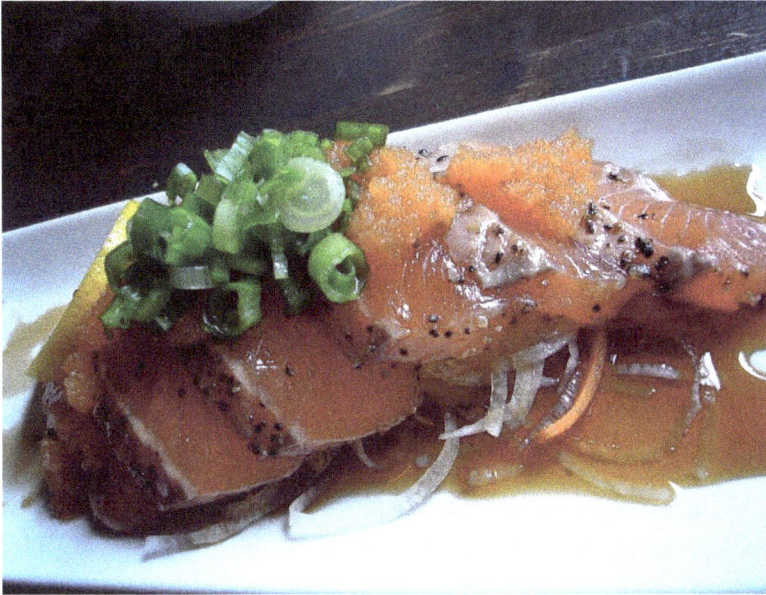

Servings: 4

Preparation Time: 105 minutes

Cooking Time: 8 minutes

Ingredients:

- 4 tablespoons of extra-virgin olive oil, divided
- 2 tablespoons of fresh lemon juice
- 1 teaspoon of ground turmeric
- 1 teaspoon of ground cumin

- Salt and ground black pepper, as required
- 4 (4-ounce of) boneless, skinless salmon fillets
- 6 cups of fresh arugula

Instructions:

1. In a bowl, mix together 2 tablespoons of oil, lemon juice, turmeric, cumin, salt and black pepper.
2. Add the salmon fillets and coat with the oil mixture generously. Set aside.
3. In a non-stick wok, heat remaining oil over medium heat.
4. Place salmon fillets, skin-side down and cook for about 3-5 minutes.
5. Change the side and cook for about 2-3 minutes more.
6. Divide the salmon onto serving plates and serve immediately alongside the arugula.

Lemony Salmon

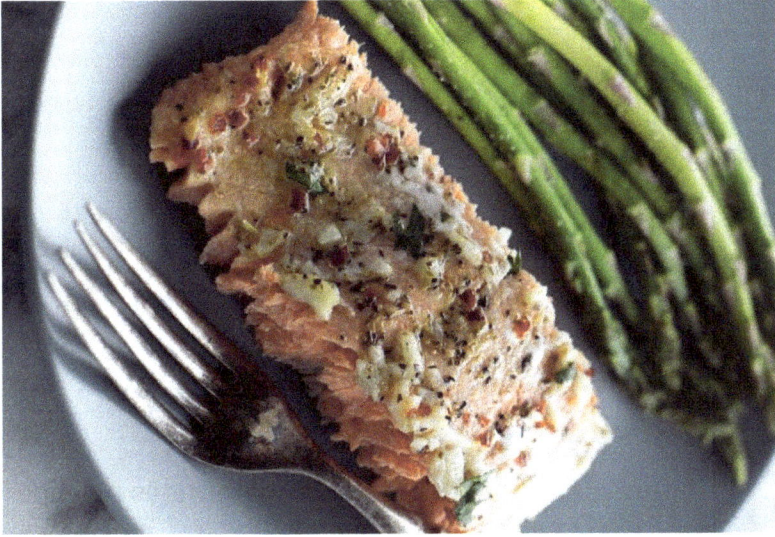

Servings: 4

Preparation Time: 10 minutes

Cooking Time: 14 minutes

Ingredients:

- 2 garlic cloves, minced
- 1 tablespoon of fresh lemon zest, grated
- 2 tablespoon of olive oil
- 2 tablespoons of fresh lemon juice
- Salt and ground black pepper, to taste

- 4 (6-ounce of) boneless, skinless salmon fillets
- 6 cups of fresh spinach

Instructions:

1. Preheat the grill to medium-high heat.
2. Grease the grill grate.
3. In a bowl, place all ingredients apart from salmon and spinach and blend well.
4. Add the salmon fillets and coat with garlic mixture generously.
5. Grill the salmon fillets for about 6-7 minutes per side.
6. Serve immediately alongside the spinach.

www.ingramcontent.com/pod-product-compliance
Lightning Source LLC
Chambersburg PA
CBHW050756030426
42336CB00012B/1842